Rommel Furst Brito
Gustavo Lucas Costa Valente
Barbara H. A. Ferreira

Bovine mastitis little discussed

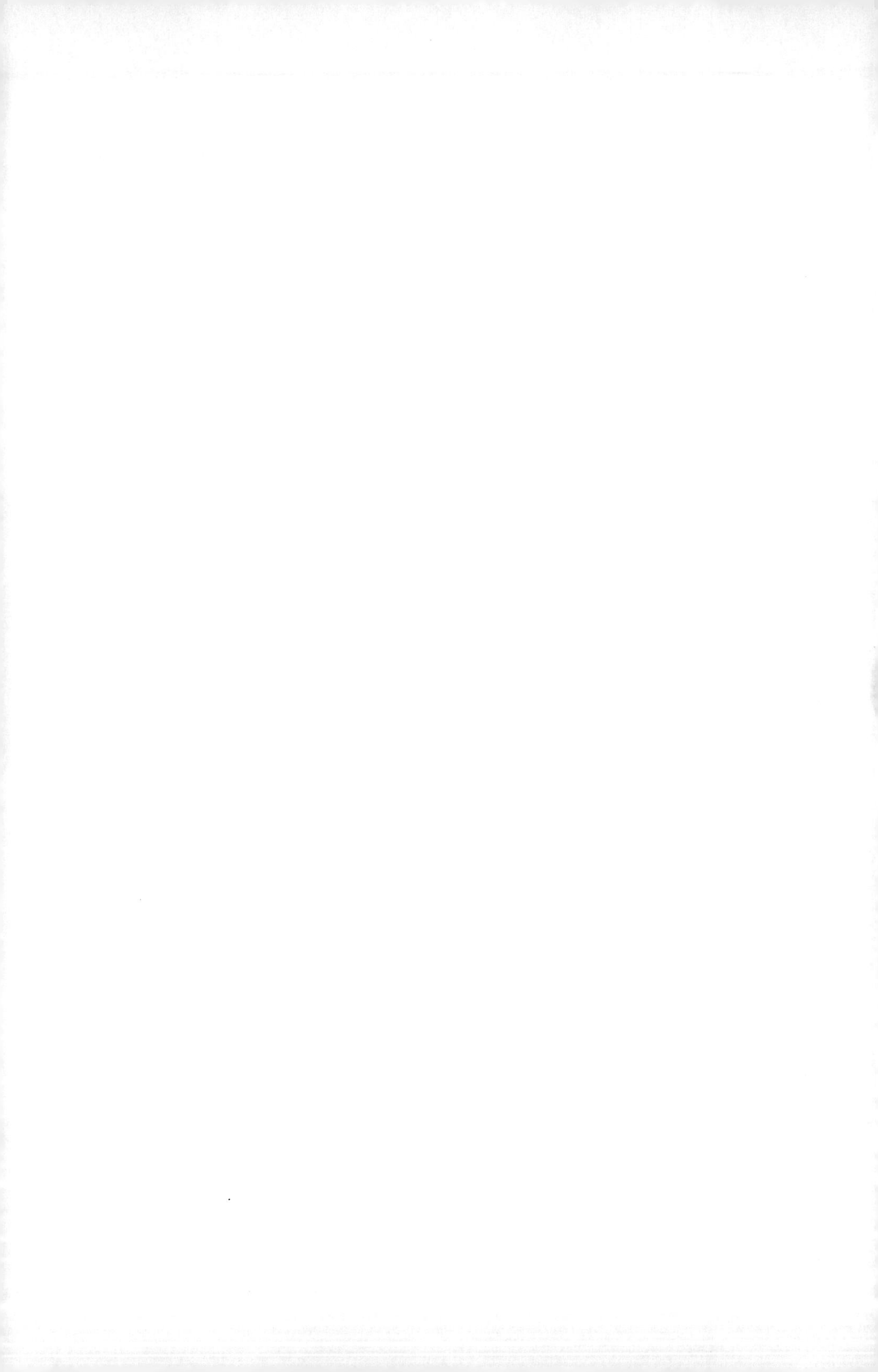

Rommel Furst Brito
Gustavo Lucas Costa Valente
Barbara H. A. Ferreira

Bovine mastitis little discussed

Literature reviews

ScienciaScripts

CHAPTER 1

Mastitis caused by *Streptococcus equi* ssp. *zooepidemicus*

Rommel Furst Brito

Gustavo Lucas Costa Valente

Barbara Helena Alves Ferreira

1. Introduction

Lancefield group C streptococci are grouped into two species, each with two subspecies: *Streptococcus dysgalactiae* ssp. *equisimilis and S. dysgalactiae* ssp. *dysgalactiae', and S. equi* ssp. *equi,* and *S. equi* ssp. *zooepidemicus* (Benítez, *et al.,* 2006).

S. equi ssp. *zooepidemicus* is a beta-haemolytic Gram-positive bacterium that belongs to the microbiota of the respiratory and urogenital tracts of horses and is the main causative agent of mastitis in mares, and is also recognised for causing sporadic cases of mastitis in cattle, goats, sheep and camelids (Pelkonen *et al.,* 2013; Las Heras *et al.,* 2002, Obied *et al.,* 1996, McCue, *et al.,* 1989). It is an opportunistic pathogen associated with a wide variety of diseases, for example pneumonia, septicaemia, mastitis, placentitis and endometritis (Rasmussen, *et al.,* 2013). *S. equi* ssp. *zooepidemicus* has already been found in healthy carriers in other species such as pigs and monkeys (Rasmussen, *et al.,* 2013), but it is responsible for respiratory disease in cats, with an outbreak in a cattery being reported by Blum *et al.* (2010), and also associated with "kennel cough" (Chalker *et al.,* 2013). The variety of species affected extends to wild animals, as demonstrated by the report of the isolation of *S. equi* ssp. *zooepidemicus* in common seal *(Phoca vitulina)* and grey seal *(Halichoerus grypus)* in the North Sea (Germany) during two outbreaks with phocine distemper virus by Akineden, *et al.* (2007).

The fact that mastitis in mares is mainly caused by *S. equi* ssp. *zooepidemicus is* corroborated by the study carried out by McCue *et al.* (1989). The authors reviewed 28 cases of mastitis in mares, and in 19 cases (71%) aerobic bacteria were isolated. Of these, *S. equi* ssp. *zooepidemicus* was the most commonly isolated bacterium, accounting for approximately 37 per cent of the total. The results found are summarised in Table 1 below.

Table 1: Results of aerobic cultures of milk samples from 17 mares with acute mastitis

Organisation	No. of isolates	% of isolates
Streptococcus zooepidemicus	7	36,8
Streptococcus viridans	1	5,3
Streptococcus agalactiae	1	5,3
Staphylococcus spp.	2	10,5
Actinobacillus suis spp.	2	10,5
Pasteurella ureae	1	5,3
Enterobacter aerogenes	1	5,3
Klebsiella pneumoniae	2	10,5
Escherichia coli	1	5,3
Pseudomonas aeruginosa	1	5,3

Adapted from McCue *et al.* (1989)

Streptococcus spp. are the second most important group of microorganisms as causal agents of mastitis in sheep, after *Staphylococcus*. Although *S. agalactiae, S. uberis* and *S. dysgalactiae* are the most frequently identified species, other *Streptococcus* species, such as *S. parasanguinis,* are also responsible for causing infections in mammary glands (Las Heras *et al.* 2002). In their work, Las Heras *et al.* (2002) described an unusual outbreak of mastitis in sheep caused by *S. equi* subsp. *zooepidemicus,* which the authors consider to be the first report of mastitis associated with *S. equi* ssp. *zooepidemicus* in sheep. The authors recorded a frequency of 4.7 per cent of *S. equi* ssp. *zooepidemicus* isolated from sheep with clinical mastitis. Although the number of cases of mastitis caused by *S. equi* ssp. *zooepidemicus is* tiny compared to other species of bacteria, the reduction in milk production and premature drying make mastitis caused by *S. equi* ssp. *zooepidemicus* a serious health and economic problem (Las Heras *et al.* 2002).

(range 5-89 years); 86.2% of the cases lived in the urban area of Monte Santo de Minas, and 16 cases in other municipalities in the states of Minas Gerais (Arceburgo, Itamogi, São Sebastião do Paraíso), Acre (Rio Branco) and São Paulo (Batatais, Milagre, Mococa, São Bernardo do Campo, São Paulo, Santo André, Ribeirão Preto, Santo Antônio da Alegria). The incidence rate of nephritis in residents of Monte Santo de Minas was 7.5 cases/thousand inhabitants. Among the signs and symptoms, the most frequent was haematuria (90.9%), followed by cervical lymphadenopathy (73.1%) and oedema (52.0%). Forty-two people affected (24.0%) were hospitalised. Of the 24 people aged 60 or over, 12 were hospitalised. Four cases progressed to acute renal failure, requiring haemodialysis, with subsequent recovery. The average time between onset of symptoms and medical attention was 7.6 days, with a median of 4 days. In the group of hospitalised cases, the average time was 11.7 days, with a median of 10 days. There were no deaths (Soares *et al.*, 2017).

Six ice-cream parlours in the municipality, which manufacture their own products, were identified as possible sources of contamination. After the Health Surveillance team took action, it was found that ice cream parlours I, II and III used pasteurised milk from dairy A, ice cream parlours IV and V used raw milk supplied directly from rural properties and ice cream parlour VI used powdered milk, duly registered. Dairy A was located in Monte Santo de Minas, received milk from 35 rural properties and was not registered with the competent bodies, having been banned by the Instituto Mineiro de Agropecuária (IMA), which raised suspicions about the efficiency of the pasteurisation process of the milk processed in this industry.

In the case-control study carried out by Soares *et al.* (2017), 32 cases and 128 controls were included, with 14 cases confirmed by laboratory criteria and 18 by clinical epidemiological criteria. Among the participants, there was a high consumption of milk and dairy products, including raw milk and milk from dairy A. In the adjusted analysis, cases were more likely to have consumed ice cream (OR=9.67/IC95%: 2.08;44.89) and milk in plastic bags (OR = 4.04; IC 95%: 1.43 - 11.47) when compared to controls

(Soares *et al.*, 2017).

Benítez *et al.* (2006) reported an outbreak of *S. equi* ssp. *zooepidemicus* infection on the island of Gran Canaria, Spain, between February and April 2003. The clinical and epidemiological study of the outbreak found 15 patients (5 women and 10 men) with a mean age of 70 years (range 47-86 years). Infection with *S. equi* ssp. *zooepidemicus* was primarily bacteraemia in 6 cases, bacteraemia associated with aortic aneurysm in 4 cases, septic arthritis in 2 cases, pneumonia in 2 cases and meningitis in 1 case. Five patients (33.3%) died. The case-control study showed that the consumption of cottage cheese made from unpasteurised milk was associated with diseases caused by *S. equi* ssp. *zooepidemicus* (OR= 4.5; 95% CI: 1.57 - 19.27).

Balter *et al.* (2000) reported an outbreak of glomerulonephritis in Nova Serrana (MG), with 134 confirmed cases, attributed to the consumption of cheese made from raw milk contaminated with *S. equi* ssp. *zooepidemicus*. Of the confirmed cases, 99 (74%) occurred between February and April 1998, and the average age of the patients was 37 years (range 6-81 years). 97 patients (72%) were hospitalised with an average length of stay of 3 days (Balter, *et al.*, 2000).

Balter *et al.* (2000) interviewed 50 patients and their respective controls and concluded that patients who consumed fresh cheese, farmhouse mozzarella and brand A yoghurt were more susceptible to the disease than controls. Of the foods, cottage cheese was the only one consumed by the majority of patients with nephritis, and 36 per cent of the patients who consumed the product reported buying it from the supermarket. The individuals consumed an average of 4 dairy products (ranging from 0-9). The frequency of cottage cheese consumption was the same for patients and controls. Three individuals (two patients and one control) denied consuming any dairy products on a regular basis (Balter *et al.*, 2000).

Brand A yoghurt came from a large industry and was distributed throughout the state foetus five days after clinical signs of mastitis appeared. *Streptococcus zooepidemicus* was isolated from the milk, but not from the foetus or placenta. The mare was febrile, with unilateral inflammation of the udder and pain to the touch, but no other signs of systemic disease.

Pisoni *et al.* (2009) reported an outbreak involving 2 of 22 lactating goats. Both goats showed local and systemic signs of clinical mastitis. The somatic cell count was high in the milk of both goats ($>7\text{x}10^6$ SCC/mL). The daily milk production of the infected goats was between 0.9 and 1.5 L before the diagnosis of mastitis and drastically reduced in the affected mammary glands, which ceased milk production 2 to 3 days after the onset of symptoms.

Las Heras *et al.* (2002) reported an outbreak involving 13 out of 58 lactating ewes (morbidity rate of 22 per cent). The cases were detected 30 days after weaning, and in a period of 2 weeks after the first case was detected, after the event no other cases of mastitis were reported. In this outbreak the mastitis was always unilateral, with no signs of acute udder inflammation, and no systemic signs. The milk took on a watery appearance, containing small clots of pus. Similar to what was reported by Pisoni *et al.* (2009), milk production by the ewes varied between 0.5 and 0.9 litres and drastically reduced in the affected mammary glands, ceasing production 5 days after the onset of symptoms. There was no mortality among the ewes, but the affected glands never recovered their milk production.

5. Control and prevention

Las Heras *et al.* (2002) warned of infections caused in species other than the mare, associated with manual milking, where contact with horses may have been the source of the infection. In the reported outbreak, a mule on the farm grazed alongside the sheep and they were confined in the same environments. Although the mule was healthy, with no recent history of respiratory disease, Las Heras *et al.* (2002) pointed out that *S. equi* ssp. *zooepidemicus* is a component of the equine microbiota, and that routine contact between species may have provided an opportunity for infection. As for hand milking, Las Heras *et al.* (2002) pointed out that the procedure was carried out in poor hygienic conditions. The milker didn't wear gloves and didn't sanitise his hands between animals, and this is a risk factor that may have contributed to the transmission of *S. equi* ssp. *zooepidemicus* from the mule to the mammary glands of the sheep via the hands of the milker during milking, as well as the spread of the disease between sheep.

Therefore, we should consider segregating production and working animal species, both on pasture and in confinement, in order to avoid exposing the dairy herd to *S. equi* ssp. *zooepidemicus,* which is a commensal of the equine respiratory and urogenital tracts. In addition, the hygienic milking procedure should be adapted, which is key to preventing the spread of mastitis in the herd, as well as the emergence of new cases, and when possible, mechanical milking should be recommended.

Pelkonen, *et al.* (2013) evaluated the susceptibility of *S. equi* ssp. *zooepidemicus* to antibiotics isolated from humans grown on blood agar. As a result, they found that the colonies of *S. equi* ssp. *zooepidemicus* isolated were sensitive to erythromycin, clindamycin, penicillin, vancomycin and cephalexin. Benítez, *et al.* (2006) evaluated the susceptibility of *S. equi* ssp. *zooepidemicus* to antibiotics isolated from human patients and identified by biochemical assays, and confirmed the findings of Pelkonen, *et al.* (2013) regarding sensitivity to erythromycin, penicillin and vancomycin, as well as rifampicin and levofloxacin. However, the samples were resistant to tetracycline and clindamycin, which contrasts with the results found by Pelkonen, *et al.* (2013).

Las Heras *et al.* (2002) also tested the susceptibility of *S. equi* ssp. *zooepidemicus* isolated from sheep's milk, obtaining measurements of the diameter of the halos for the following antimicrobials: penicillin (36 mm), amoxicillin (36 mm), amoxicillin associated with clavulanic acid (35 mm), tetracycline (9 mm), streptomycin (12 mm),

S.; GARCÍA, A. G.; ANTÚNEZ, I. A.; MAROTO, A. S.; RIVERO, M. B. Outbreak of *Streptococcus equi* subsp. *zooepidemicus* Infections on the Island of Gran Canaria associated with the Consumption of inadequately Pasteurised Cheese. *European Journal of Clinical Microbiology & Infectious Diseases, N.25,* p.242-246. 2006.

BLUM, S.; ELAD, D.; ZUKIN, N,; LYSNYANSKY, L; WEISBLITH, L.; PERL, S.; NETANEL, O.; DAVID, D. Outbreak of *Streptococcus equi* subsp. *zooepidemicus* Infections in Cats. *Veterinary Microbiology,* v.144, p.236-239. 2010.

CHALKER, V. J.; BROOKS, H. W; BROWNLIE, J. The association of Streptococcus equi subsp. zooepidemicus with canine infectious respiratory disease. *Veterinary Microbiology,* v.95, p.149-156. 2003.

CONTRERAS, A.; LUENGO, C.; SÁNCHEZ, A.; CORRALES, J. C. The Role of Intramammary Pathogens in Dairy Goats. *Livestock Production Science,* v.79, p.273-283. 2003.

KE, C.; QIAO, D.; GAN, D.; SUN, YL; YE, H.; ZENG, X. Antioxidant Activity *in vitro* and *in vivo* of the Capsule Polysaccharides from *Streptococcus equi* subsp. *zooepidemicus.* Carbohydrate Polymers, v.75, p.677-682. 2009.

LAS HERAS, A.; VELA, A. L; FERNÁNDEZ, E.; LEGAZ, E.; DOMÍNGUEZ, L.; FERNÁNDEZ-GARAYZÁBAL, J. F. Unusual Outbreak of Clinicai Mastitis in Dairy Sheep Caused by Streptococcus equi subsp. zooepidemicus. *Journal of Clinicai Microbiology,* v.40, n.3, p. 1106-1108. 2002.

McCUE, P. M.; WILSON, W. D. Equine Mastitis - A Review of 28 Cases. *Equine Veterinary Journal,* v.21, n.5, p.351-353. 1989.

OBIED, A. L; BAGADI, H. O.; MUKHTAR, M. M. Mastitis in *Camelus dromedarius*